If You Have Gray Hair...**BEWARE**

Tips, Tools and Tricks
to get
Your Needs Met in Healthcare

Ebie Andrew

ISBN:1511418753
ISBN-13:9781511418751

This book is dedicated to my beautiful wife, Leah who is
my greatest champion.
And also to Jules Myers and the Red Barn Institute for
showing me I already knew the way.

CONTENTS

Introduction   i

1   Why Beware?   9

2   Whose Responsibility is it Anyway?   13

3   The Doctor Visit   21

4   The "My Healthcare Notebook" System   29

5   Emergency Services   32

6   Legal Documents   38

7   Caring for Someone with Cognitive Impairment   42

8   Facilities   47

9   Alternative and Complementary Medicine   63

10   Insurance   66

11   Staff   69

12   Notebook Layout   72

Acknowledgements

There are more people to thank than there is room on this page, however a few people contributed in enormous ways, I cannot thank you enough.
Leah, for everything.
Jules Myers for beginning my process and providing the encouragement to seek my passion! Patte LeVan for your countless number of edits and suggestions. My Mom, for listening and using the tools I gave her and giving me invaluable feedback. My Dad for proofreading, encouragement and suggestions. For my brother Frank, for telling me to live boldly.

INTRODUCTION

This book is written to assist those older people, and those who care for them, who use the American healthcare system. Much of the information in this book is applicable to other healthcare systems in the world.

The American healthcare industry is a for-profit industry designed to make money. It is also a service industry, although administrators usually want you to forget that.

The American healthcare industry makes money by you being ill or injured or in some way needing their products and services. Fortunately this is a frequently occurring state in the course of being human, so business is steady. In order to increase the profit *margin*, the companies have to decrease either quality of products or services, or get you to think you need *more* products or services. Notice profit margin, not just profit. Profit is how much money a company makes (sales over costs). Profit margin is the percentage of profit over costs as a whole.

How do you get what you need and want in an industry that **you** need, but that wants to make the biggest profit they can from your need?

How do you keep from being convinced to purchase products and services you do **not** need when the people you trust are telling you it would be best?

How do you hold that industry accountable for what it does to you?

The people who are working in the industry **and** making the *least* amount of money are the people who are in the industry usually because they are born caregivers and want to help people be well. These people have been educated in the industry of healthcare. These are the people you interact with; nurses, therapists, and aides, etc. How do you help these people to help *you* get what *you* need and want and protect yourself at the same time?

It is my fervent hope that this book will help you to acquire the type of care that you want and need from the American healthcare system.

Chapter 1

WHY BEWARE?

Ageism in the American healthcare industry--a word of caution.

Ageism: definition - prejudice or discrimination against a particular age-group and especially the elderly.

Our society's dominant culture supports many "ism" behaviors even when they are not intended, and are often perpetuated by people who are not aware they are doing it.

I have gray hairs. I earned every one of them. I feel that people who have survived long enough to get gray hair deserve some respect for that accomplishment; however it also is a way in which our society marks people as "old." The altered treatment you get from that label is ageism.

In my 20+ years in healthcare, I have met only a handful of people who did not harbor some level of ageism. Even if they exhibit no signs or symptoms of any other isms, they have ageism. It is everywhere in our society and no place more prevalent than in advertising. Most advertising targeting older persons in our society is created to tell them they should not look act or feel old and that being old is the worst thing they could be. There are infinite numbers of products to help us not look like older persons, or to convince us to get medications or services so as to not feel like older persons. Or in the worst case, to convince us that we are old, and therefore vulnerable, and more old and vulnerable than we really are, then scare us into spending our money out of fear of what will happen to our old and frail selves.

The amount of money spent on advertising to the elderly is amazing! Most of the advertising is time spent convincing you that you should live in some level of fear. Then telling you how you can spend money to not be afraid or so that you won't look or feel old. The elderly in this country are being bombarded with phone solicitations and flyers in the mail and television, advertisements ad nauseum. If you have an older parent, try ordering something for them on the internet and have it mailed to your home. You will be amazed at the stuff you will get selling things to seniors. Everything from medications to senior dating services!

In the healthcare industry it is mostly the pharmaceutical companies that are advertising, but senior living places have recently gotten into the game in very big ways. Be very wary of anyone, including your healthcare people, who say they are offering something to you or that you have to have something because you are seniors. And if they use a generality, such as "people in your age group" or some other nonsense, beware! This shows that they are not thinking of you as an individual, not taking your particular circumstances into consideration, and are attempting to plug you into a generalization. If for any reason you think that they might be selling something you really do want or need, take 24 hours and talk to someone you trust about it. Ask yourself this question "Am I purchasing out of a fear that I have not had before?" If your answer is yes, beware, they may be selling you false security for a baseless fear.

For quite some time there was a company that was trying to convince everyone that they should use a scooter and Medicare would pay for it! That they would be safer, have fun, and infinitely more freedom! Many of those scooters or power wheelchairs ended up in basements or closets as the people they were given to were not even instructed in how to use them. That company is out of business now and getting service for those products has become a nightmare for the people who do use them.

Another thing to think about: the healthcare industry is telling us that the "baby boomers" are all coming of an age where they will need care. Really? I do not think it is true that just because you age you become ill or debilitated. I do think that the pharmaceutical industry would like you to think that you need their drugs and that you will continue to need them for the rest of your life.

I have known several 90-something-year-olds who are driving around doing what they please including golfing and joining clubs. I am seeing people get older before they need assistance and even older before they have health problems. Not everyone has health problems. However, as humans we often encounter periods where navigating the healthcare system is necessary and the tools outlined here will help.

I do know that the baby boomer generation is the last of the people who have retirements that were not traded or gambled on the market, but built on solid promises by companies that used to keep their commitments to their employees. The baby boomers are now considered "seniors." In many ways these are the people with the most "disposable" income in this country. The marketing people of every industry know it and want to get as much of it as possible. Marketing people also generally believe that the seniors are easily convinced to spend that retirement. Make sure that the spending you are doing is not out of fear of what **might** happen, but out of need or for your enjoyment.

In addition to all the direct ageism, there is also a lot of subtle and often infuriating ageism. Like the 20-something who calls you "honey." Or when you are out with your adult kids and they ask the "kid" if you want something to drink. These are just small things that let you know they are not seeing you as a fully functioning, contributing member of society.

Call them on it.

Tell the waiter to ask you, not your kid. Tell that sweet young thing to use your name, or ma'am or sir, but show some respect.

It reminds them that you are still in full control of your faculties. I am not saying you have to be mean about it, but just let them know they were not being respectful. I guarantee that 20-something who just called you honey would not call the next 20-something to walk through the door "honey" in that condescending tone of voice, and they should not do it to you either!

Chapter 2

WHOSE RESPONSIBILITY IS IT ANYWAY?

Your doctor is not responsible for your health.

You are.

The D in doctor does not stand for deity. I am going to say this a lot.

This may come as a surprise to some of you. The doctor is only responsible to help you manage your disease processes **and** to help you manage your symptoms in the ways that he/she has been trained to do, usually with pharmaceuticals.

It is sometimes difficult to realize that you are responsible for something that you have always looked to others to take care of. The healthcare industry will not be held responsible for your health, just for treating your illness or condition.

If you do not take responsibility, I assure you, no one else will.

Disease processes: this means any diagnosis that is

1. not temporary and
2. will in the course of time be progressive or require monitoring or intervention to prevent, or manage, the symptoms of progression.

A fracture will become a history of fracture when it is healed, most bacterial infections can be cured, but many diagnoses cannot be cured, only "managed."

What we are talking about here is the diagnoses that will need to be treated, watched, or otherwise monitored and that you expect to have for the rest of your life. Examples include: arthritis, chronic obstructive pulmonary disease (COPD), congestive heart failure (CHF), cancer (CA), Parkinson's, or any other thing that the doctor feels should be monitored and/or treated for the rest of your life.

There is a VERY big difference between maintaining health, and disease management or symptom control. Most doctors and other western medicine (allopathic) healthcare professionals are not trained to maintain your health or even counsel you on how to do this. They are trained to manage your symptoms and control the disease processes through pharmaceuticals.

The D in doctor does not stand for deity.

The doctor does not know what is happening in your life, does not know what is happening with your health...unless *you tell him/her.* Doctors are not responsible to keep you healthy. Many of them are in the business of selling you pharmaceuticals or procedures. Sometimes doctors do this because of the risk of litigation, sometimes because they were told to, often by pharmaceutical companies, sometimes by the very insurance companies that are paying your bill. For example: I cannot tell you how many times I have seen a person be discharged from the hospital and no one thought that they were ready, but the insurance company has a limit on how long the patient can stay in the hospital based on the diagnosis, not on the patient's well-being.

Another example is when they are released from the hospital and now they are on far more medications than ever before. Some of them they need, or needed while in the hospital, some not so much. No one is in the business of trying to take you off these medications unless you request it or the medication is obviously causing problems. If I ask you why you are on (for example) a cholesterol medication, you say you did not know you were. You may also know that you have never had high cholesterol before in your life and have not had any cholesterol tests that you were aware of. Not only are there other ways to bring cholesterol down than medications, but I have seen the medications have nasty side effects. Patients often do not remember if anyone told them or talked to them about the options or that they even needed the medication, **if** they needed it.

The follow up appointment with your primary care physician is for this purpose. *You may well need the medication, but it is the responsibility of the healthcare professional to educate the patient and the responsibility of the patient to ask as many questions as needed to know what they are taking and why.*

The D does not stand for deity.

WE DO NOT UNDERSTAND EVERYTHING ABOUT HOW THE BODY WORKS!

The doctor understands **a lot** about how the body works and how medications can help. If we understood why people get arthritis we would stop it! Most doctors do what they can to maintain your function as best they can though pharmaceuticals. There are more things that we do **not** understand than there are things we do know about how the body works. Western medicine resolutely does not look at anything that is not repeatable, demonstrable, and peer reviewed. This is especially true if there is a risk of litigation, or a decrease in the faith of the public in the healthcare professional or in the industry as a whole.

Most of the research being done in healthcare is on new drugs and procedures to make money for the pharmaceutical and medical equipment supply industries. It is very hard to find information on where the monies come from for research, but all the information agrees that most research is funded by private industry for a future profit. If there is not a product goal, meaning to develop a specific product like medication, the research is up to organizations like the NIH (National Institute of Health) which is primarily funded by the government--which means our tax monies--and private donations and nonprofit foundations which usually contribute to very specific research only. At a time when so many budgets are being cut, this is one of them. Please do not take my word, look it up, the internet is a wondrous thing.

We do make progress in understanding every year. Research monies are very limited for things that are not pharmaceutically based. But research and understanding of how our bodies work does progress yearly and every year that you can keep yourself healthy is another year of understanding that may bring cures for, or education to prevent, many diseases and conditions.

There has been a huge drive--mostly by Medicare, although **all** insurance companies seem to follow Medicare's lead--to hold the hospitals and the doctors responsible for your health. They are now denying payment if you are re-hospitalized for the same diagnosis within 30 days of having been discharged with the same diagnosis, at least for *some* diagnoses.

This is a fail.

The hospital and their doctors are not responsible for your health after discharge.

You are.

It is your behavior, just plain circumstances and many other factors that will determine your chances for readmission. But this is how Medicare keeps from paying the hospitals and so saves money.

It is about the money.

It is also another way to tell people they are not responsible for their health. It is a lie. You are responsible for your health. Your choices and genetics and toxins and many, many other factors, some of which we do not even know yet, determine your health. You are the only one in charge; you are the only one who can make the decisions that affect your health, and the more hospitalizations you have the higher your risk for long term health issues.

You are responsible for choosing your doctor.

Your doctors are your employees. You hire them to do a job.

You want to pick ones who have the same basic philosophies that you do. If you are a strong believer in diet as a way to manage your health, do not pick a doctor who thinks that what you eat does not affect you. If you are a person who thinks that pharmaceuticals were designed to be taken so that you can eat the way you want and live the way you want, do not pick a doctor who thinks you need to eat healthy. This is the most important step in being happy with your healthcare because no matter what service or specialty you need, your doctor will refer you to practitioners of like mind, unless there is no option, as in a very rural community.

This goes for all your healthcare employees.

When you are looking for a healthcare provider,

always ask people who have had experience with the service you are looking for. If you need an orthopedic surgeon, ask the physical therapists at the nearest physical therapy clinic which doctor's patients rehab the best. They will tell you. They want good outcomes for their clinic and will tell you who they think does the best job. Ask respiratory therapists about pulmonary doctors, and the dialysis clinics about the renal doctors. Be aware when calling a clinic for referrals that if it is owned or affiliated with any doctors in particular, you may get a prejudiced answer--but you may get a totally honest answer too. If it is owned by a group of doctors, you might want to call a second clinic as well.

I have often recommended looking at the first visit with your new doctor as "the interview" for you to decide if you will hire that doctor. You should take a list of questions to the first visit that will tell you if the doctor shares your philosophies or not. You may wish to consider giving your opinions and observing the doctor's response, or just asking questions. Here are some sample questions:

1. Do you feel that medication is necessary to good health after the age of 65?

2. Will you provide education about why you are recommending either a medication or procedure or a referral?
3. Do you feel that most health concerns can be addressed with diet and exercise?
4. Will you be as concerned about the quality that I want for my life as the quantity?
5. How frequently do you refer to specialists?
6. Do you feel that all tests should be completed at the ages recommended no matter what state the health of the person is that you are ordering them for ?
7. Do you take the monetary cost and the side effects into consideration when prescribing, or just the efficiency of the medication?
8. How do you feel about complementary and alternative healthcare?
9. How available are you if I have an urgent need/Do you take "emergency" appointments?
10. What method do I need to use to contact you? (i.e. phone or email)

Think about when you have had an urgent need to get in to see the doctor, but did not feel that an emergency room visit was appropriate, and ask the doctor how the office staff is instructed to handle those situations and make sure you are okay with that.

Think of times that you have had treatment in a doctor's office that you felt was really the best. Figure out why you felt that way about that visit and tell the prospective doctor what you value in treatment and see how s/he responds.

Think of the times you did not feel well treated, why you felt that way. Check to see how the staff are treating other people who are there to see this doctor, and consider whether you would want to be treated that way.

A good doctor will have good staff that are generally happy to work there. If there are a lot of "new" staff, or if the staff seem particularly stressed or the atmosphere is strained, it could be a sign of bigger problems. When staff are required to consistently perform in an environment that is less than optimum for a long period, it is certain mistakes will happen. This often happens when administrators try to save money or increase the profit margin by doing the same or more work with fewer staff or inadequate equipment.

A high-demand low-satisfaction work environment in healthcare means danger for the patient.

Beware of places that readily and frequently tell you they are "short staffed" or "understaffed." It is much safer for the patient if they say "so and so left (insert reason here) and we have not found the right replacement yet."

The quality of the office décor does not reflect upon the quality of the doctor or his staff!

In my experience, the really quality care clinic is not as concerned with the appearance as they are the happiness and health of the patient.

Chapter 3

THE DOCTOR VISIT

When you do find a doctor or other health care professional that is a good fit for you, do not make the mistake of thinking that they know everything or that what they recommend is law.

The D does not stand for deity. Doctors are not omniscient. You need to tell them what is going on and give them as much information as possible. One of the most important things you can do, not just for yourself but for your doctor(s), is to keep a notebook. The next chapter is an entire chapter on how to build your healthcare notebook.

Before visiting your doctor, make two lists. The first should list everything that you think would be important for the doctor to know. The second should list the things that are not as important but that are related. Add any questions that you may have about your healthcare to the list of related items.

For example, if you have diabetes and you notice that since you have switched to using xylitol as a sugar substitute your blood sugars have been lower, in the first list you would write that your blood sugars are lower and the date that started, and in the second list when you started using the xylitol. We will go into more detail on this in the notebook chapter.

Then make two copies of both lists. One for the doctor and one for yourself, keep yours in the doctor visit section of the notebook.

You do not know what the doctor might think is important. When the **doctor** enters the room - not the assistant, not the nurse, *the doctor*--hand him/her one list and say, "I brought this for you." You will be happy because five minutes after leaving the doctor's office you will not think "Oh shoot, I forgot to mention...." and your doctor will be happy because s/he will have all the pertinent information in a short list and can ask questions as s/he thinks of them. As the doctor goes over the list you can make notes on your list in the notebook and check off the items as they are addressed. This is also time efficient for the doctor; keep in mind that the doctor has about 10-15 minutes for the entire visit, so if you cannot get through the list, make another appointment. Or when you do make an appointment, ask for two back to back appointments to address different issues. This keeps both of you from frustration and meets both your needs. Just keep in mind that if you have a copay, you will have two copays for two appointments.

If you are seeing a doctor for a specific issue e.g.: your hip, and after the surgery or other treatment you are now experiencing knee pain, you need to make an appointment for your knee, not just ask the doctor to address the knee during a follow-up for your hip. The insurance companies all frown on this and it can be troublesome for your doctor.

The D does not stand for deity. Just as they are not able to know anything that you do not tell them, likewise not everything they recommend will be the right thing.

Do you feel like a "guinea pig" when the doctor prescribes medication? In a sense you are. No two people are the same. Although your doctor may know what "family" of medication you need, s/he has no idea which one will work best for you until you try it. Some of the medications will be eliminated due to your particular history of sensitivity or allergic reactions. Some because they are not compatible with something else you are already taking. But it is your feedback that guides your doctor to the right medications for you.

It is all the information you give to your doctor that helps him or her determine which medication is best. Sometimes it really is just down to trying them and seeing what works best. You are the one who decides what works based on the report of improvement or lack thereof to your doctor.

Your doctor is responsible for picking the treatments that will help your conditions, but you have responsibilities to the doctor as well.

You are responsible for:

1. Making sure that all the questions are answered
2. The insurance cards are presented
3. The information requested is given
4. To keep your appointments
5. Cancel appointments as needed with reasonable notice
6. Ask any questions that you have
7. Say if you do not understand the directions or the explanations you have been given.
8. And report any progress, problems or side effects due to the medications or other treatments as soon as you are aware of them.

Tell them what you want and need. Listen to those you trust. **Ask as many times or ways that you need to be able to understand what they are telling you**. It is your responsibility to be sure that you understand what is happening with your health.

Be very sure that **if** you allow someone to make decisions for you in your health care, in your finances, in any way, that they are someone who will follow **your** wishes, not do things their way, but **your** way.

Your healthcare employees are responsible to give you their professional opinion, and to make sure that they have explained in a way that you can understand their recommendations. That is all. Just because "the doctor said" is NOT a reason.

You are responsible for your own health!

The doctors can only give you a recommendation. It is a professional, educated recommendation and they do have a responsibility to recommend only things that will not harm you; however you are the one to decide if you want to take their recommendations. "Do no harm" does not necessarily mean that what they recommend will actually benefit you, or be the best option for you.

If you have done your homework in choosing

your healthcare professional, then it would be a good idea to take their advice.

If you find that you have doubts about their advice on a regular basis, or you feel they are not listening to you, talk to them about it, give them a chance to explain or change how they serve you. If they do not listen, or do not change their behavior, and you are still having issues with that healthcare professional, fire him/her and hire someone else.

I know that it is easier said than done when looking for someone who will take your insurance and fit with your philosophies, but it is well worth the effort if it is possible.

Always, always get a second opinion for anything that is "serious." Meaning serious to *you*. There is no reason to not get another opinion. Especially when you are not completely comfortable with the recommendation or diagnosis. You should always go outside the practice and preferably to a totally unconnected practice for a second opinion if possible. In rural areas and difficult situations, this may not be possible, but it is best to try. This is a responsibility on your part to care for your health.

Having said that, not all insurance will pay for a second opinion, however if you have concerns it will cost you more in pain and suffering if you are right than what a second opinion will cost you in money. As of the writing of this book, Medicare will pay for a second opinion *only* for what they consider an elective surgery such as a total hip or knee replacement.

Always, always, always research every recommendation. In this day and age of the internet, it is totally irresponsible to not do your research. If you do not have access to the internet, go to the library.

Serious unashamed plug for your local library. I love them, they are the best resource for researching anything! If you do not know how to navigate the internet, the library staff does and will help you or sign you up for help, or help get you to a class. This is important.

Never, never take a medicine if you do not know what it is and what it is for and why the doctor prescribed it. Then when you know all of that, ask the pharmacist about it. When you have done that, look it up on the internet. When you leave the doctor's office you should know if you have a prescription, why you have it, what it is for, what it will do, what side affects you should watch for and how long you will be taking it. And what things you can do, if anything, to not need the medication in the long run. You are responsible for your health, and you need to know. If you are not able to, have a family member or friend who is willing to do the research and inform you.

It is okay to leave the doctor's office without prescriptions!

I have had the experience of meeting people who felt that if the doctor did not give them a prescription then the doctor did not do the job. This is also the medical industry's standard assumption of how the patients feel. This is ridiculous. Doctors should only be prescribing when it is needed. You should be very happy if the doctor says you do not need a prescription! It means you are doing a good job maintaining your health! That is your job!

If you get prescriptions, you would do well to ask what you can do to improve your health so that you do not need the prescription. Every pill has a price to your body in side effects. For example, we now know that antibiotics exact a high price in your gut health, they do not cure viruses and can even decrease your immune response. Many drugs that are overused are also causing unintended side effects in our communities as well. The overuse of antibiotics coupled with incomplete instructions or people who did not follow the instructions have created "superbugs" like MRSA (methicillin-resistant Staphylococcus aureus) and VRE (Vancomycin-resistant Enterococcus). Both are antibiotic resistant bacterial infections.

Doctors are frustrated with the healthcare system too. They are no longer able to doctor the way they would like to for several reasons--litigation, education, insurance companies, pharmaceutical companies, legislation for political reasons - the list goes on.

Doctors have a limited amount of control in their practices now. The insurance companies determine how many patients a doctor should see in a day. They do this by negotiating the amount they will pay the doctor so low that they need to see many patients to make a profit. At this point a doctor needs to see one patient about every 10 minutes, maybe less depending on how many insurance networks the doctor has been able or required by the practice to "sign on" with. It is one of the reasons doctors are leaving the field. That and being told what they can and cannot say or prescribe in their own office with their professional opinion. It is a problem, and one I do not have an answer for, but you can ask the questions and make it clear to your doctor and your insurance company what you want. There is power in numbers, but only so much energy in a day and the companies count on you and your doctor to just accept what they tell you.

The last thing I have to say about the doctor office visit is about respect. It is an important part of the relationship you have with your doctor. Not only do you need to be able to respect your doctor, but the doctor and her/his staff need to respect you too.

Your time is just as valuable as theirs. You need to be on time for your appointments, but they do too. If you have made an appointment for say 11 a.m. and they are not getting around to seeing you until 12:30, this is not respectful. Please be understanding if your doctor does this only on occasion and the staff explains that your doctor does see patients on an emergency basis, as that may be you needing the emergency appointment some time. If this becomes a regular occurrence every time you go, consider billing the doctor's clinic for your time, or just finding another doctor.

Chapter 4

THE "MY HEALTHCARE NOTEBOOK" SYSTEM

I have developed a system to maintain control over your various health issues and manage your healthcare staff. It is called the "My Healthcare Notebook."

It should be a 3-ring binder preferably, and we will discuss all the things that go into it in the different chapters of this book. In the back of the book there will be examples as well to give you a visual idea of what it should look like.

In the front of the notebook keep an up to date medication and supplements list that includes everything, even over-the-counter medications (OTC), vitamins, herbals, all of it. This should be kept in a protective plastic sleeve. At the top of this page, list all the drug and food allergies that you have. If you do not have any allergies that you know of, you should write that here as well. Make sure to add even the temporary medications like mucinex or robitussin if you have a cold. If you leave empty lines in the hard copies, you can pencil them in with a start and stop date so you do not have to print a whole new list every time some little thing changes. It is best to keep three copies, one for yourself, one to give to emergency responders if needed, and one for the health care appointments you have.

In the same protective plastic sleeve, just behind the medication list, should be copies of your DPOA (durable power of attorney), living will, and/or Advance Directives (we will discuss these in another chapter). As well as a list of all your current physicians and their phone numbers and a list of your diagnoses.

You will want a page just after the plastic sleeve to track any of your vitals that you monitor. Examples are: Blood pressure, weight, temperature, pulse, oxygen saturation rates, blood sugars or any other thing you check regularly.

You will want a page that lists the medications and how many times a day you take them and then gives you room to check them off as you either take them or fill a medication box.

Make sure that you have a separate section in your notebook for each of your healthcare providers. If you are a caregiver for another person, keep a separate notebook for yourself and one for the person you are caring for. If you have several specialists or different types of healthcare professionals that you see, keep a different *section* of your notebook for each specialty and then let each of them know what is going on with the others. Keep each section in the same notebook so you can refer different healthcare employees to what others have said. This will also allow you to know who said what and in chronological order. Keeping all of your healthcare professionals apprised of all of the changes to your care is important, especially your primary care physician (PCP) who is like a head chef in the kitchen. They keep an eye on what everyone else is putting into the "pot" i.e., you.

There is another added benefit to the notebook that although I hope you will never need it, is good to know about. If you keep the notebook religiously and date everything as it happens, it could be pivotal in a court of law if the need should arise. There is a common saying in the healthcare industry: "If you didn't write it down, you didn't do it." This is used during training of staff to encourage them to document anything that is "billable" in order to make as much money as possible. It also has unintended side effect. If they did not write that they did something they shouldn't have done, it is difficult to prove they did it. If you are keeping the notebook updated and writing down everything with the date, and if you are in the hospital, times as well as dates, it will be admissible in a court of law just like a journal. In a hospital setting, this is invaluable.

Keep a separate section if you have home healthcare providers coming into the home so they can write down or add to your notebook any instructions or recommendations that they have for you, and you can write down anything you need them to know.

Please see the back of the book (Chapter 12) for a full layout of the contents of the "My Healthcare Notebook."

Chapter 5

EMERGENCY SERVICES

Before we go any further, make sure you have a Durable Power of Attorney (DPOA). All people over the age of 18 should have one.

A DPOA is a person who can make healthcare decisions for you in the event you are not capable of making those decisions. If you have any strong beliefs in how you wish to be or not to be treated, make sure your DPOA knows it and has agreed to uphold your beliefs, even if they do not hold the same beliefs.

Your DPOA needs to be someone who lives close to you and can respond in case of an emergency. The fact that you have a DPOA and who it is should be on your person at all times. In your wallet or in your purse, keep a card that says DPOA and list the name and contact information of your DPOA. You may want to laminate it. On cell phones, in your contacts, make an ICE (In Case of Emergency) contact and make this your DPOA. DPOA forms can be obtained free of charge from the Area Agency on Aging in your area, or from several sites on the internet. Just put in the search box "where can I get free DPOA forms" and hit the enter key. We will discuss this more in the next chapter.

Patient Advocate

The person no one talks about and everyone should have is a patient advocate. Some healthcare facilities have one on staff. They are, however, hired by the facility and their primary loyalty is to the job. You always want to have an advocate. It would be best to have someone identified as your advocate before you need one; this should be your DPOA if they live close, but if not you will need someone who can be there very quickly.

You are not in any condition to self-advocate when in a healthcare facility such as a hospital or rehab unit.

Your patient advocate must be someone you trust who is able to question authority, fight for what you want and get answers to your questions and results to your requirements!

Generally when there is an emergency you are not thinking very clearly. You just want whatever is causing the emergency to stop. You go to the ER to get someone knowledgeable to be in charge, someone that can tell you what is wrong if you do not know and fix it.

The Emergency Room

How do you know what method to use to get there? In an emergency, if you or the person with the emergency is not able to get themselves into a vehicle to go to the emergency room (ER), call 911. It is what they are there for. It is better to wait for the EMTs (emergency medical technicians) to show up and identify the most urgent needs than to try to get someone to the ER yourself, especially if the emotional stress is high. If they feel that the patient should not go to the ER and you do, insist. They will take the patient to the hospital. However, if there was no emergent need, you may end up with the entire bill for the emergency medical transport service and it can get quite expensive.

If you are going to the ER to get someone to fix whatever is wrong, you will be disappointed. This is not how the ER works anymore. The ER is now more about triage than it used to be. Triage means: is it bad enough to be admitted? If not they will make recommendations and maybe a referral to your PCP or a specialist and send you home. If you are of the Medicare generation (anyone 65 or older) it is not even triage anymore. Medicare has stopped paying hospitals if they readmit a person within a certain number of days with the same diagnosis that they were treated for on their last admission. This means that if you are discharged from the hospital with CHF(congestive heart failure) and you are back in the ER within a certain amount of days (the number changes year to year), Medicare will not pay the hospital for your stay. This means they will not admit you if at all possible.

Beware: Medicare does not pay for "observation." You need to ask, "Am I being admitted?" If you are not, ask why you are not being sent home, if it is not enough to admit you, then they need to:

1. Send you home with instructions on what to do to not be in a situation where you need to come back
2. Tell you what conditions warrant returning to the ER, and
3. If you end up back at the ER within a few hours to a day in worse shape, then they need to agree to admit you.

Questions you should be able to answer before you leave the ER are:

1. What are the parameters outside which I should come back, or bring my loved one back to the ER? I.e.: blood pressure over 180/100, or pulse over 125, temperature over 104f?
2. What medications am I leaving with?
3. What are the medications for and what should I watch for in the way of side effects or adverse reactions?
4. Am I being referred to a specialist and has the ER given me that doctor's information?
5. How can I care for myself or my loved one to prevent coming back to the ER?
6. If you do not understand, ask! Then ask again and again until you are sure you know what they are telling you.
7. It never hurts to get the instructions in writing. They will give you papers, but if an instruction is given verbally and not written down, do not hesitate to ask them to write it out. If the verbal instruction is different from the written one, ask them to change the written instruction to match the verbal instruction.

They do not want you to come back--not as much as you do not want to be there--but still, they want you successfully home.

If they give you an answer that seems "not right"

question it. I actually know a lady who took her mom to the hospital when she was very ill. They sent her home and told the daughter that her mom would be safer at home where she would not be exposed to additional infections.

Really?!

So they are admitting to not being able to prevent the spread of infection inside the hospital? It is true that it does happen, but it is their job to prevent the spread of infections and there are guidelines set forth by the Center for Disease Control (CDC) and the state Department of Health. They are called standard precautions and everyone should be using them all the time. The risk should not be higher than in the home. That person took her mom home, and ended up back in the ER the next day much worse. This time they did admit her. But she may never have gotten worse if they had admitted her the first time.

ICU

Another mention here is the ICU (intensive care unit). Most people do not realize that the job of the doctor on the unit is to not allow "that body" to die on his/her shift. That is it. There is no real consideration for the patient's future quality of life, just don't let them die on "my watch." Unless there is a legal DPOA (durable power of attorney) with the required paperwork and a living will that spells out what the person wants, the staff will do whatever it takes to keep the body alive. Everybody has different desires and requirements about what they want. I have had people choose to die of infection rather than allow amputation of an unsalvageable limb. I have also had people who want every possible measure taken to maintain life in a loved one who is in the end stages of a terminal and painful disease process. Only you can decide and you need a DPOA and a living will (see next chapter) to make your wishes known and respected.

Only you know what you are comfortable with so when you choose a DPOA, make sure that it is someone who will follow your wishes, not their emotional desires.

Urgent Care

If you have insurance that is not Medicare, it is often more economically reasonable to go to the Urgent Care; however make sure that you do not have an emergent need. The wait in the Urgent Care can be just as long as in the ER and if you have an emergent need, you may have to go to the

ER and start all over.

Chapter 6

Durable Power of Attorney, Power of Attorney, Guardianship,

and Living Will

DPOA or Durable Power of Attorney, is the legal instrument, or document, that gives another person the authority to make healthcare decisions for you **only** in the event you are not able to make them for yourself. From here on I will use the term DPOA to refer to the person that the document gives this power to. Everyone over the age of 18 should have one. As soon as you are 18 years old, your parents do not have as much right to say what will happen in your care as the doctor does, and could legally not be given information about you.

This is also handy for those times when your loved one is sick enough that they really are not able or willing to make a decision. Most times the doctor will ask the family what they want, but if at any time the family wants something other than what the doctor feels is best, if the family does not have DPOA, their wishes may not be followed. If you have a DPOA there is less likely to be a fight, and legally the DPOA gets to make the decisions.

PA or Power of Attorney gives legal power to a person to perform financial or legal business dealings for another person. This is very important if you need someone else to go to the bank or the department of motor vehicles or any other number of things for you. You should have someone delegated to this role in the event you are not able to make these decisions or execute these responsibilities.

Guardianship can only be legally assigned by a judge in a court and only if you can prove that the person you wish guardianship of is not capable of understanding the consequences of their choices. It is difficult to obtain if the person has never needed one before, but is very important if they do need one. This takes away the right of a person to make decisions for themselves and places all of the responsibility on the guardian. Even if the person is able to respond appropriately, it is only the guardian that is allowed to make decisions for the person legally. It is a very heavy responsibility and not to be entered into lightly. Other people will be monitoring the guardian's decisions and abuse is sometimes open to interpretation.

A note about the importance of deciding what you want and do not want prior to an emergency.

Aside from religious beliefs, there are personal comfort levels and just plain reasonable accommodation and convenience. Know that if you are at home, there are services to help you. You must pay for these services. If you are in a facility there are costs, and they will help you, but they are there to make money off of your needs.

Discussing these things ahead of time, knowing what your family can and cannot do, knowing what you are willing for them to do for you and not do for you is important. If you need help toileting, or showering, are you willing for your children to help you with that? A stranger? Can you afford help in the home? These are things that can mean a difficult conversation with family, but worth it. We will talk more about difficult conversations with family in the next chapter.

Living Will or Advance Directive

A Living Will is a declaration of what a person does or does not want in terms of medical care. It can be confusing and uncomfortable. It is important to have if you have strong feelings about what you do or do not want in the event that you have a serious medical event that could require drastic measures to prevent death. Everyone has a different comfort level.

I have known people who would rather die than be placed on life support systems. I have also known people who want to be kept alive no matter what, even on life support as long as possible no matter the circumstances. Nothing you want is right or wrong, but you will probably not get it if you do not tell people what you want ahead of time.

Advance Directives are the same things as Living Wills.

All of these documents, with the exception of Guardianship, are available from your local area agency on aging, several websites, most hospitals and the local department of health.

Make sure that the forms you get are the correct ones for your state.

Copies of these forms, completed and signed by the correct people--including the doctor in the case of advance directives--should be in the front of the healthcare notebook, preferably just behind the medication list.

See the back of the book (Chapter 12) for the full layout of the healthcare notebook.

Chapter 7

CARING FOR SOMEONE WITH COGNITIVE IMPAIRMENT

If you suspect cognitive impairment or mental health issues:

The only way to address an issue is to first identify it. Then you can find out what you can do about it. Like everything else, your doctor could be an ally. When you have done the work to pick a doctor that is of the same philosophies, you can talk to them about it and trust they will guide you in a direction that will be agreeable to you. This is no different when it comes to emotional difficulties, or if you are caring for someone else who is experiencing these issues and you need advice.

If your car broke down and you had the basic skills to repair it, you would go to the auto parts store. You would get the tools and the parts you need, maybe some direction. If you take those things home and put them under the couch, your car will not get fixed.

Likewise, if you have cognitive issues, getting to a professional that can give you the tools and the advice you need to make things work for you is essential. But you have to use the tools. Just as in your physical health, you are responsible to use the tools.

Unlike other facets of healthcare, mental, emotional and cognitive issues require hard work on your part to make them stable and functional. Even if they never work again the way they used to, for example after a stroke, compensation techniques can make cognitive, mental and emotional issues at least functional if the damage will not heal.

There is no magic pill for anything!

Especially in this area of health.

If you are thinking your loved one is having cognitive difficulties, it can be much harder to help them than if they have physical ailments.

This is the hardest thing for some people to admit to and to face. If your loved one is making decisions that you really think are not what they would have wanted just a few months or years ago, or seem to not be able to make decisions that have good long term consequences, it is time to have a very difficult and honest discussion with that person.

He or she may be confusing times or events, may have "unreasonable" anxiety, or try to cover their confusion with humor or anger. Whatever behavior it is that makes you think that your loved one is having cognitive difficulties, I cannot stress enough how important it is to talk about it and not just blow it off. The consequences of medication errors and driving judgment errors can be fatal.

It is best to start by asking why they are making the decisions they are making. What is their thinking? Let them know that you are interested and that you know you will be facing the same decisions as you age. If they are not able to give coherent reasons, or if they become confused or defensive, tell them what you would do and ask if they would like you to help them or even do some of the decision making for them. Be absolutely honest. This is your parent/wife/husband. They know when you are hedging or outright lying! They can always refuse to allow you to help, but please try. It reduces regret.

There are cognitive tests that can help people to know where the deficits are, if there are any, then skills can be offered to compensate for the deficit so the deficit it is not impairing that person's function. Speech therapists and some occupational therapists specialize in this type of therapy. If you feel it is needed, discuss it with your doctor as a prescription is needed for most of these services to be covered by insurance.

If you feel that *you* may be having memory or cognitive issues, **do not cover it up**! Talk to someone. Your doctor, family, a friend. It may be embarrassing, but the earlier the detection and diagnosis the easier it is to treat. That goes with all ailments, but most especially cognitive and memory loss issues. New and very exciting treatments are being developed all the time. Do not wait.

If there *is* a diagnosis of cognitive impairment:

If you are caring for someone who has some type of dementia or other cognitive impairment, they may not be able to tell you the things that the doctor needs to know. As the caregiver, you will need to try to identify the changes and report these to the doctor as a third party. This is difficult and often not attended to by the healthcare professional as it ought to be. If you are the primary caregiver it is likely that you know the patient better than anyone else.

Changes in routine and environment can precipitate changes in cognitive ability in the later stages, but in the earlier stages, challenge to the thought processes is really beneficial. Even if it takes a long time, it is worth it to write down the things that you notice for the care staff you engage with.

Example scenario: Dad starts with the occasional complaint that his arm hurts in the morning, not every morning, but it is getting more frequent and when he goes to the doctor the doctor asks him if he has pain and he says no. This is reasonable to him because he does not have pain *now*. If you have been keeping his notebook, you can tell the doctor that he has complained of pain in his arm six mornings out of the last ten. If you are tracking the changes to his environment you may notice that you changed his pillows one week prior to his first complaint. At this point, the doctor may recommend massage therapy or physical therapy to decrease the pain while you return his pillows to the previous type. This can save both of you a lot of pain and suffering later as the symptoms worsen and more intervention is needed to control the pain.

There are several types and levels of cognitive/mental impairment, and it is always best to allow the patient to take as much responsibility for their own health as possible. If they can make the entries in their healthcare notebook, then encourage them to do so.

When the dementia or medication needed creates a situation where it is no longer safe for the patient to drive or make their own decisions, someone needs to be honest enough to tell the patient. Make sure that when you are ready to "take the car keys away" that you let them know it is done with love, that you fear for their physical safety and the safety of others.

Sometimes it is impossible to make this painless. Some of the patients become very angry and defensive. It is often best when this happens to recruit your healthcare staff, as it can be easier for the patient to hear and take in from a professional rather than from family.

Having said that, even a doctor is not allowed to tell a patient that they are not allowed to drive; doctors can only recommend. The Department of Motor Vehicles can revoke a person's license. But that does not keep them from physically driving if they have access to a vehicle and the keys.

The very last resort is to call Adult Protective Services. It is an option and they are there to help.

Their ability to assert power changes from state to state. In some states they have the power to remove a patient from a living situation if there is obvious abuse, physical, emotional, mental or financial. In other states only in the case of physical abuses, in some states no power to remove the patient at all. They are, however, a good resource and have the training to provide information at the least.

Chapter 8

FACILITIES: HOSPITALS, SKILLED NURSING, ADULT FAMILY HOMES AND ASSISTED LIVING

The first thing I want to address with all facilities is the Patient Bill of Rights. Upon admittance to any of these facilities you should receive a copy of the Patient Bill of Rights.

READ IT! KEEP IT! REFER TO IT OFTEN! Here it is in its entirety as it is written on the federal government website:

BILL OF RIGHTS ADOPTED IN 1998 BY THE U.S. Advisory Commission on Consumer Protection and Quality in the Health Care Industry:

Information for patients

You have the right to accurate and easily-understood information about your health plan, healthcare professionals, and health care facilities.

If you speak another language, have a physical or mental disability, or just don't understand something, help should be given so you can make informed health care decisions.

Choice of providers and plans

You have the right to choose health care providers who can give you high-quality health care when you need it.

Access to emergency services

If you have severe pain, an injury, or sudden illness that makes you believe that your health is in danger, you have the right to be screened and stabilized using emergency services. You should be able to use these services whenever and wherever you need them, without needing to wait for authorization and without any financial penalty.

Taking part in treatment decisions

You have the right to know your treatment options and take part in decisions about your care. Parents, guardians, family members, or others that you choose can speak for you if you cannot make your own decisions.

Respect and non-discrimination

You have a right to considerate, respectful care from your doctors, health plan representatives, and other health care providers that does not discriminate against you.

Confidentiality (privacy) of health information

You have the right to talk privately with health care providers and to have your health care information protected. You also have the right to read and copy your own medical record. You have the right to ask that your doctor change your record if it is not correct, relevant, or complete.

Complaints and appeals

You have the right to a fair, fast, and objective review of any complaint you have against your health plan, doctors, hospitals or other health care personnel. This includes complaints about waiting times, operating hours, the actions of health care personnel, and the adequacy of health care facilities.

Consumer responsibilities

In a health care system that protects consumer or patients' rights, patients should expect to take on some responsibilities to get well and/or stay well (for instance, exercising and not using tobacco). Patients are expected to do things like treat health care workers and other patients with respect, try to pay their medical bills, and follow the rules and benefits of their health plan coverage. Having patients involved in their care increases the chance of the best possible outcomes and helps support a high quality, cost-conscious health care system.

Other bills of rights

This bill of rights focuses on hospitals and insurance plans, but there are many others with different focuses. There are special kinds, like the Mental Health Bill of Rights, hospice patient bill of rights, and bills of rights for patients in certain states. Insurance plans sometimes have lists of rights for subscribers. Many of these lists of rights tell you where to go or whom to talk with if you have a problem with your care.

The American Hospital Association has replaced its bill of rights with a patient care brochure. You can find that online here;

http://www.aha.org/advocacy-issues/communicatingpts/pt-care-partnership.shtml

Each facility and each state has their own bill of rights. Make sure you know them.

I have worked in every one of these type of facilities and for the most part the people working in them are trying to do their jobs in a good way. Do keep in mind however, that all of these facilities, whether they are nonprofit, for profit, secular, religious, private or public are there to profit from your care needs. Sometimes the desire of the staff to do good work can conflict with the organization's desire to make money or at least avoid litigation. While this is not always the case, you need to beware. Particularly in the hospital, you are more than likely not in good enough shape to self-advocate. I hope you are, but be sure to have someone who can advocate for you. (See chapter 6).

One of the most common abuses of patient rights occurs when the patient feels they are ready to go home. If the patient is in full control of their cognitive faculties or the family knows they are able to care for the patient at home and wishes to take the patient home, but the facility personnel say the patient may not go: **This is not okay.** Often the facility representative says something along the lines of "the doctor/therapist has not released you yet" or "we have to wait for the doctor/therapist approval."

No, you do not. The facility is your employee; *you* decide when the job is done.

Insist that they get everything ready for you to go. Pick a day, tell them to make sure that the pharmacy knows your needs and that you will be leaving, and their job is to assist you in making a successful transition home. That is what you are paying them for.

They may threaten you with "AMA" or leaving against medical advice. Do not worry, all the medical professionals can do is advise, they cannot compel you to comply with their wishes to get more money out of you.

If they are still insistent that you cannot go, ask them if they are imprisoning you against your will. Then call the ombudsman. Any person in any facility will be able to get this name and number for you and in most places it is required to be publicly posted.

Under the federal Older Americans Act every state is required to have an ombudsman program that addresses complaints. They often work through the offices of the Area Agency on Aging. They are there for any facility including hospitals.

Please be sure to do your homework before entering any healthcare facility!

This is a good link for Medicare rules, options, and what is covered: **www.medicare.gov**

Talk to the people who live in the facility if it is a residential facility. Take an unscheduled tour. Eat a meal if it is a facility where meals are provided. If you do not like the food, it will not matter for very long how much you like the people.

Check out the hospitals in your area, if there is only one and you do not like it, make sure that you let your DPOA know that if you have to go to that hospital in an emergency, you wish to be transferred to the hospital of your choice as soon as is possible.

Hospitals

This is the link to a booklet from the Department of Health and Human Services about Medicare and hospital stays and can be very helpful: **www.medicare.gov/Pubs/pdf/11408.pdf**

I have earlier addressed the fact that the only thing the medical professionals can do is recommend. Most doctors believe their viewpoint is "the correct" viewpoint and will argue with anyone, even other doctors about it. You are the one to decide what will happen to you and whose advice you wish to listen to.

I know of a situation in which a person was in the hospital and the doctors who shared the shifts disagreed on pharmaceutical treatment. Every new shift, the doctor who came on duty changed her medication. It got to the point where she was not able to understand what was going on and she kept getting worse. Her granddaughter who did not live near her was a nurse and came to visit. She found out about the several medication changes and put a stop to it. The granddaughter was able to decide which doctor's recommendation she thought was reasonable for her grandmother and the patient was home in three days.

Most hospitals are using contracted "hospitalists." Hospitalists are doctors who specialize in working in the hospital and do not have a practice anywhere else. These doctors often rotate floors in a hospital or rotate regions in a "health system," or just rotate to whichever hospital the company they work for has a need for a doctor. It is not that these people are not good at their jobs, many of them are very good, but there is no vested interest in the community. You will not get a follow-up appointment with that doctor, and indeed may never see them again as they are rotated to a different region or state. This is not to say that you will in any way receive less care. You should remember that your relationship with this doctor will likely be for the duration of your stay only.

There are a great many people in the hospital at all times. Staff, patients, administration, volunteers, visitors, contracted workers. There are so many opportunities for mistakes that it is mind boggling. The staff do everything they can to decrease those chances. Please have patience when the 4th or 5th person asks you your birth date and full name and then checks your wristband. They are trying to make sure you do not receive Suzy-down-the-hall's medication or procedure. The number of people who have been in the bed that you are occupying in the last month is sometimes amazing.

On the other hand, because there are a great many people in the hospital and fewer staff than there are patients, it is up to you to demand what you want.

If the nurse walks in and does not wash her hands, ask her/him to.

Do not be shy about your safety!

They may have just washed their hands walking out of the last person's room and used hand sanitizer on the way to your room and if you do not see them do it, feel free to ask them to wash up! This is your life and we have created too many superbugs to not take extra precautions.

While you are in the hospital, have your

notebook with you. Ask the names of the doctors and nurses and write them down. Or ask someone else to write it down, or ask them to sign in and out of your room. Make a note of every change in your treatment, who ordered it and when the change took place. Note all the results, positive and negative. This information will help the doctors to help you as well as providing you with a way to hold them accountable for their actions should you need to.

Keep track of all the tests, test results, and procedures that you experience while in the hospital. If you are not capable, ask your advocate or DPOA to do this for you. Recruit your community (visitors, pastor, friends, etc.) to get your notebook and bring it to you or purchase one in the gift shop for you if you went to the hospital in an emergency and were not able to get your notebook. It will be worth it.

As an advocate for someone else, keep a notebook for yourself as well as the patient. Include who told you what about the patient's condition or diagnoses or testing and when. If you think it is important, write it down. It is very difficult to remember details two weeks later when the bill arrives or the patient's doctor wants to know something.

Keep track of anything that seems to be "not right" by writing it down in a section by itself.

If someone working in the hospital is particularly good at their job, or more attentive to you, make sure you tell their superior. It matters. Really, one word of appreciation for good service is the way to get it to happen again!

If you have been in the hospital, always get a follow up appointment with your PCP (primary care physician) as soon as is possible after your discharge. If you have done your homework to pick a PCP, then your doctor has your history, and with any luck knows you and your preferences. This is very important when it comes to the changes that the hospital makes to your medications while trying to get whatever brought you to the hospital under control. Those medication changes should not stay the same once whatever it was is under control or you will end up with other problems.

If the hospital says that you may not go home, that you have to go to a skilled nursing facility for rehab, remember that they can only make a recommendation. I have had people who had kids and grandkids who were perfectly able to care for them at home and the doctors did not feel that it was enough.

It is still your choice! If the doctor does not want to sign your release due to his/her professional opinion, that is okay. You can still go home. I wish to encourage you to think about it and talk to the people who will be providing support for you at home. Make sure that they are able to provide the support you will need to be successful at home and not end up back in the hospital. Remember that things will NOT be same when you return home as when you left.

I also suggest that you offer a compromise to the doctor and request home health. If you can do that, there will be an RN and other professionals with their eyes on you at least within a few days of your being home and probably regularly for the next few weeks.

Skilled Nursing Facilities (SNF)

This link will take you to a PDF download of a booklet provided by the Department of Health and Human Services for Medicare and Medicaid stays in a SNF:
www.medicare.gov/Pubs/pdf/10153.pdf

You may know them by their more common name: Nursing Home, although they are calling most of them Rehab Centers now.

You need to require a certain level of care to be admitted to a skilled nursing facility or SNF. Medicare will not pay for your stay at a SNF unless you qualify. The requirements to qualify change, but for at least the last 20 years *one* of the requirements is that you have a three night stay in the hospital. That is three consecutive midnights. It is important to know that three days is not sufficient and the SNFs are expensive. If you are admitted to the hospital at 2am, you have not been there one day until you pass the next midnight, even if you were in the ER since 5pm the previous day because you had not been admitted until after midnight.

Medicare pays for the first 20 days of a qualified stay 100%. For the next 80 days at 80%. The SNF will try to keep you there as long as possible. I repeat the above paragraph:

One of the most common abuses of patient rights occurs when the patient feels they are ready to go home. If the patient is in full control of their cognitive faculties or the family knows they are able to care for the patient at home and wishes to take the patient home, but the facility personnel say they may not go, **this is not okay**. Often the facility representative says something along the lines of "the doctor/therapist has not released you yet" or "we have to wait for the doctor/therapist approval."

No, you do not. Really.

Even if you leave against medical advice or "AMA," you will still be able to get services in your home if you wish. Many places may try to tell you that if you leave AMA you cannot. That is not true. You can.

On the other hand if they try to give you just 48 hours notice that you *must* go home, that is also not legal. They must give you two weeks and allow time to prepare for your coming home. They may say that you have reached your potential and that Medicare will no longer pay; that is also illegal. If you have reached your potential, they still have to cover you for the two weeks to get ready to go. This is Medicare law.

I want to caution people here that if you have been in the hospital and then a rehab center or nursing facility, when you go home it will not be as easy as when you left. If you are not able to drive, I suggest you request home health services and if you can drive, outpatient therapy. More on that later.

Everything that applied to the hospital applies to

the SNF. The need for an advocate can be much greater here, but there are more options if you are not happy with the services.

Assisted Living Facilities (ALF)

These are the places that can give you the right amount of support without you having to give up your independence. They usually have several levels of care with each level of increased care costing more money.

Most of these places are large, with several floors and more than one dining area; many have activity departments and group outings and transportation services to medical appointments. There are also smaller places with one dining room and fewer residents if you would prefer a quieter building. However, they are expensive, and without the correct type of long-term care insurance are often impossible to afford.

Some have restrictions on visitors, so if you have grandkids who fly in from out of town and stay with you for a few days, make sure that is allowed. Some will give you assigned parking spaces, but have no place for visitors.

Some places have contracts with outside services like home health agencies for therapies. Make sure if you have services you wish to continue after you move into a facility, that those services would be allowed to follow you to the facility, or that you are willing to switch companies to one that provides the service in the facility you are moving to.

Adult Family Homes (AFH)

These are excellent alternatives to the assisted living facility or the skilled nursing facility. Be as cautious with these as with any other facility.

AFHs usually have only a few residents, usually fewer than six, and are located in neighborhoods in a large home and are staffed around the clock with an aide. The better ones are staffed with CNAs (certified nursing assistants). All of them have an RN who visits regularly, although it varies from state to state how often that is required.

These types of facilities usually admit patients who have a higher care need than ALFs, but some are good at transitioning a person back to the home. Most people who are in AFHs are living there and no longer have another home.

As with any other facility, talk to the people who live there, not just the staff.

Home Health

Home Health is a service that is very good to have if you are going home instead of the rehab unit after a hospitalization. It is a service that is complimentary for people in the home environment or the AFH, or the ALF. It provides Skilled Nursing Care, Social Services, Physical Therapy, Occupational Therapy, or Speech Therapy as needed to help patients return to their homes but still receive services to improve their condition and help them be as independent as possible in the home environment. This is a VERY underutilized resource and provides wonderful benefits. The professionals in the facility settings such as the hospital or rehab unit cannot address the challenges you will have at home, as they do not know what your home or daily lives are really like.

My next door neighbor entered the hospital for a total hip replacement, then to a SNF for rehab. During her stay at the SNF the therapists asked her how many steps into her home. She told them just one small step about 4 inches. She and her husband have lived in that house more than 30 years. They built it themselves, every beam. The step into the house is between 8 and 10 inches. She really did not believe it was that high until she got home and was astonished. She has gone up and down that step for 30 years, but never thought about how high it was because it was not a problem before.

Home health helps you to make your environment functional to your abilities and improve your abilities to function in your environment with minimal adaptations.

Medicare part A covers this service and there are qualifying conditions, so not all people returning to the home will qualify.

These people are a very good resource for equipment needs, services, as well as many other things.

Outpatient Services

This can be anything from Lab work to Imaging to Therapy services. If you are able to get out of your home to a vehicle, get into and out of the vehicle without assist, tolerate the ride to where services are provided, and participate in the service and get home without a considerable or taxing effort, outpatient is for you. The outpatient clinic has equipment that cannot be brought into the home. The goal of the Home Health professional is usually to get you to the point that you are able to get to the outpatient clinic where "the good toys are"!

Those Infernal Surveys

So, want to know about those infernal surveys that everybody sends you?

In the interest of saving money, the surveys are sent out so that the facilities and service providers can be ranked. Those not in the top 95% of the nation have money withheld on services provided. Not to mention, wouldn't you look for the highest ranking service provider? The rankings really do not mean anything; they are solely for the purpose of saving money.

The only thing that counts is the highest possible score, so for instance, if the scale is 1 – 5 with 1 being lowest and 5 being the best, any number that is not a 5 counts *against* the facility or service provider. And there are strict rules that the service providers and facilities and all of their employees are not allowed to fill them out for you, tell you the scoring weight, or assist you in any way to fill them out.

If you get these surveys and you wish to give the facility or service provider a good rating, or even anything that is not a bad rating, give them the highest possible score. If you want to give them a bad rating, anything other than the highest rating will count against them.

This goes for most of the industries out there, not just healthcare. If someone asks you to please fill out their survey, ask them how the scoring is weighed!

If you want to know what people really think of the service provided, ask for testimonials from former customers and clients.

Chapter 9

ALTERNATIVE AND COMPLIMENTARY MEDICINE

There are more types of alternative and complementary medicine than I can go over in this chapter. Indeed that would take an entire new book and at least a year of research. However, let me say here that all people are different and you do not want to exclude any type of treatment that may be beneficial to you. I recommend trying everything because just like the allopathic (pharmaceutical) doctor, you will not know what works for you unless you try it. I also want to be clear that not everything works for everyone. You will be the best judge of what is right for you.

If a non-conventional (read non-pharmaceutical) practice is used **together with** conventional/allopathic(pharmaceutical based) medicine, it's considered "complementary."

If a non-mainstream practice is used **in place** of conventional/allopathic medicine, it's considered "alternative." Some of the more common types of complementary and alternative medicines are:

Naturopathy, chiropractic, massage, homeopathic, supplements, BioEnergetic Synchronization Technique (BEST), Reiki, herbal therapy, Chinese medicine, nutritional, acupuncture, yoga, meditation, exercise, journaling, mind-body, energy or crystal work, some people include the rehab therapies such as physical therapy, occupational therapy and speech therapy, etc.

The most important thing to say about this is that as long as you are living in a physical body, you are a package deal. Anything that affects your physical, emotional, mental, or spiritual self WILL affect all the others.

We are aware now that when we lose a very close loved one such as a spouse, we are at a 300% greater risk of heart attack within the first six months following that loss. Our emotions affect our physical selves. Ask anyone with high blood pressure!

It is important to try all of the things that you are comfortable with and find what works for you. Just like pharmaceuticals, you will not know what works best until you try it!

I recommend talking with people who are like-minded with you and see what they have tried. I always recommend word of mouth for promotion of the people who are really good at whatever they do.

The internet is very valuable for this type of research. Not only can you find out what any type of alternative or complementary medicine is, but you can find sites that will tell you where practitioners are and some groups who will discuss their experiences with the types of treatments as well as the various practitioners.

Keep the results of your trials in your notebook so that you can revisit the ones that worked for you and not repeat the ones that did not. Although, just because it did not work with one practitioner, does not mean that it won't with another!

In this area as well as with allopathic medicine, or Western medicine, there are few places that you can go to see if there have been complaints against the practitioner. The state department of health website and the licensing agency in the state in which you reside should have online access to search for practitioners and the complaints lodged against them and whether their license is in good standing. The Better Business Bureau is also a good resource.

Word of mouth is always the best for good recommendations and you can always ask your medical staff for referrals; they will never refer you to someone who they have not heard good things about.

Chapter 10

INSURANCE

A very short word about insurance.

Read the fine print!

Most insurance that is secondary to Medicare is called Medicare supplementary insurance and it will cover whatever Medicare covers and that is all. If Medicare covers the item or service, but pays only 80%, the secondary will pick up the other 20%. This is important if you need medical equipment.

There are a lot of things that Medicare will not cover that *if* you need them, you **really** need them! Such as adaptive equipment to help you bathe yourself. For example: If you have had a hip replacement and have restrictions such as not being able to bend at the hip past 90 degrees (very common) you will need a long handled sponge to reach your feet, and probably a bath bench or chair. Our lovely U.S. Senators passed legislation years ago that states that bathing is a luxury!

Medicare will not be covering that type of equipment. Thank you Congress! Please excuse the sarcasm.

Long term care insurance (LTCI)

Be aware of the small print. Read all of it. Be careful of bundling of services. Check to be sure that in order to receive the benefit you don't need to have very skilled services. It does not make sense to get LTCI that will only pay if you need help with bathing and dressing but will not pay for medication management. If you are in a position to need help with bathing and dressing you will probably need help with managing your medication.

Medication management is one of the most important needs! I cannot imagine having a LTCI that will not pay for this service, but they are out there!

Also be aware of what type of facility qualifies as long term care. You want to be able to use your benefit in whatever setting you need.

Know the qualifiers. Do you have to need assistance with two activities of daily living (ADLs)? Does cooking count as an ADL?

Know how many years your benefit will pay. You

want a minimum of two years and preferably four years.

Beware of the waiting period! If the waiting period is longer than the benefit pays, you are in trouble.

There is always a delay in billing with LTCI. The insurance will not pay the bill until after the service is rendered; however the facilities will bill you in advance for the month, just like rent. You need to cover the cost with the facility and get a reimbursement from the insurance company. Sometimes the LTCI will only process the claims every three months so you will end up covering three or four months before you get your reimbursement. This will get up into the tens of thousands of dollars.

Do the math. Will you pay in premiums more than they will pay out within 5 years? That is a losing deal.

Chapter 11

STAFF

Each company, clinic, facility, and lab that you do business with is your employee. You pay the companies that hire the people that do the interaction with you. These are the people who are your staff.

The staff of the companies that you hire are also your staff. They are the ones who will actually understand your needs, desires and requirements.

Remember that these are the people who got into health care because they are primarily born caregivers and they want to help people.

Health care is a very emotionally charged profession for all of the people who work "in the field." The healthcare **industry** does not care about the staff in the field. They do not value experience or ability. They value a license that can do the job for the least amount of money so as to extract the highest profit margin (see introduction). This sounds callous, but it is true.

The greater the experience and the expertise, the fewer mistakes and the better the care. The less likely there will be mistakes or someone will miss something.

If the company is aggressive in the profit-seeking area, the staff will be stressed, turnover will be high, and the care will suffer. Many companies look at staff as disposable and replaceable. Health care is a very high emotional stress profession for caring people and yet they receive little to no vacation, sick leave, or personal time. If the job itself is also for a company that has no respect for the staff, the added stress of just being on the job is high. This is a recipe for serious mistakes.

You do not need that especially at a time when you are not capable of advocating for yourself!!

The field staff have also been trained. They have been educated and trained by the industry in order to perpetuate the industry. The big pharmaceutical companies donate large amounts of money to medical schools, research at medical schools, etc. If you have any questions about this I suggest a Google search, the number of articles on the "Big Pharma" taint on the quality of medical education in this country are plentiful.

This does not mean that everyone who goes through school hands in their brain to the establishment, but many do.

If you are in agreement with these philosophies then please make sure that you have hired the companies who have staff that will direct you in that way.

If you are someone who is not in alignment with the pharmaceutical agenda, make sure that the people you are interacting with know it, respect it and will support you in making your own decisions.

Regardless of your philosophies and those of the staff, please remember that they are all your staff.

You hired them to do a job.

If they are not meeting your needs and requirements, PLEASE tell them!

If you have told them and they are still not addressing your concerns, fire them and hire someone else.

Keep in mind that if you have done your initial homework in hiring, then it would be a good idea to take the advice of the professional that you have hired. Especially if they have proven to give the kind of care you want and you are getting information you do not like for the first time. **Just because they tell you something you do not like is not reason to fire them.**

Remember that the staff are human and they have bad days and good days and most of them will be doing the best they can in a very emotionally charged profession with fewer resources every year.

If you are able to address concerns that you have with the CEO of the company, especially if the situation is one that you have previously found very beneficial and is now not--due to a change in the policies or in the ownership of the company--you would do not only yourself but everyone else a service. CEOs need to hear from the customers when things are being changed for the worse. The field staff have very little say in the workings of the healthcare companies. People without any field experience or training are making decisions that affect your healthcare safety.

Chapter 12

"MY HEALTHCARE NOTEBOOK" LAYOUT

A three-ring binder is best, but use any notebook you have.

In the front have a plastic sheet protector, in that place your medication list. Behind that: facing the opposite direction so you can read it, but in the same protector, a list of your diagnoses and your doctors' names and contact information. You may wish to have two copies of each so that you can give one to emergency responders should the need arise.

Have a second plastic sheet protector behind this one with copies of your DPOA and advance directives.

The first section should be for your use in recording any of your vitals that you monitor either daily or weekly such as blood pressure, pulse, temperature, blood sugar, weight, activity level, etc. I would also keep a checklist here for filling your med box if you use one, or taking daily medication. No matter how good your memory there will always be a day that you say "Did I take those today, or was that yesterday?" If you use a checklist to check off the med as you take it out of the bottle to either put it into the med box or to take it, you will be able to go back and know. I advocate use of the med box even if you take only two supplements. It is just easier.

The second section should be for your PCP (Primary care physician) visits. This is where you keep the information you wish the doctor to address and where you write down the things you want your doctor to know. Examples include: response to medication, any new concerns you have noticed, questions regarding how to improve your health to not require medication, if you have tried complementary medicine and how that is working or any other thing you think may be helpful.

 There needs to be as many other sections as you have specialists, or healthcare practitioners of any kind including complementary/alternative medicine, therapists, clinics, labs or any other healthcare profession you utilize.

You will need a section for emergent and hospital experiences. Even if you are fortunate enough to not ever need it, you should have it just in case. There is a sign in/out template for all your healthcare staff, but it is especially useful in a facility, and I would highly recommend using it in a hospital.

The following are examples of the templates you can download and print for free at grayhairaware.com

Monitoring Vitals

DATE	VITALS								

Medication List

	Date

Allergies:

Medication name	Dose	# Taken	Time	Start Date	End Date	Notes

Medication Name	Time of day Taken	Date Medication was Placed in the Medbox or Taken												

Sign in and out for caregiving staff

All Caregiving Staff:

Please sign and date that you were here

Date/Time	Name

My name is Ebie Andrew and I have worked in the healthcare industry as a licensed Physical Therapist Assistant for more than 20 years.

In that time I have worked in hospitals, nursing homes, outpatient clinics and in home health. I spent six years in Skilled Nursing Facilities and spent three of those years as a Rehab Director. That is where I learned quite a bit about how the type of care provided drives the profit.

I spent the last 12 years working in the Home Health industry. Each year my visits became longer, with my first visit often taking over an hour as I educated my clients in not just physical therapy, but how to manage all the different demands of their healthcare needs. It was during these visits that I became painfully aware of the lack of education available to the general public on how to manage their healthcare.

As the speed with which the industry continues to change increased, I came to realize how crucial this information was to each person I interacted with. And so the birth of this book and the personal healthcare management system I call My Healthcare Notebook.

ABOUT THE AUTHOR

Ebie Andrew lives in Washington state with her wife Leah and with their animal family that includes horses, dogs, cats, chickens and one parrot. They have three grown children and 1 grandchild on the way.

When she is not with the horses, Ebie enjoys her time exchanging information with others on a variety of topics and likes to work with art in many different mediums.

www.ingramcontent.com/pod-product-compliance
Lightning Source LLC
Chambersburg PA
CBHW070828180526
45168CB00002B/775